# Paleo Superfood Cookbook

50 Quick and Delicious Recipes

I0438941

# *Disclaimer*

This e-book is the property of the author and any publication, whether mechanical or digital, needs to be first authorized. This includes photocopying, digital printing, Xerox and all other forms. The author has taken all necessary measures to provide accurate information, however any changes in facts or figures at a future date are unforeseeable and thus subject to change.

This e-book is for educational purposes only and should be taken as such. The author takes no responsibility for any damages incurred due to the misappropriation of any of the contents stated in this e-book.

# <u>What You Will Find</u>

Paleo diets have become increasingly popular due to their various health benefits. Whether you are looking for an effective diet plan or a healthier living style, Paleolithic diets have something to offer everyone. A healthy diet incorporates all the necessary proteins, vegetables and fruits and that's what a paleo diet offers. There is no better way to opt for a healthier lifestyle than to go back to the basics and observe the diet patterns of eras gone by.

1. This e-book offers complete meal plans for people looking to adapt a paleo diet including quick and easy recipes for breakfast, lunch, snacks, dinner and desserts.

2. Each recipe comes with serving sizes, complete nutritional information including calories, carbohydrates, proteins and fats.

3. The e-book also offers valuable information of adopting a Paleolithic diet, including what is and is not allowed, how to adapt a Paleolithic lifestyle and how to stock your pantry aptly.

4. This e-book is more than a 50 recipe handbook for your kitchen, it is a complete guide to help you adapt to the healthiest and one of the most popular diet plans available. Your health story starts here.

# Table of Contents

# Introduction

In the simplest of terms, paleo diet refers to an eating style adapted from back in the day. Way, way, way back from the days when men used to live in caves, or more suitably the Paleolithic times.

So what this means is, you don't necessarily have to give up on any particular form of food, you just need to steer clear of processed food items as much as you can and make a few changes to opt for healthier alternatives when making your favorite food items.

With a paleo diet you don't necessarily have to spend time counting calories or starve your body, you can eat as much as you can and whenever you want, provided you follow the guidelines. Paleo diets have become increasingly popular since they were first introduced in the late 70's due to their easy adaptability and use of healthy and mostly organic food items.

# Benefits of a Paleo Diet

Everyone adapts a paleo diet for different reasons, results and experiences. Following are a number of benefits that a paleo diet can offer you:

## I. You Eat Real Food

This might sound like a bit of an exaggeration. But if you have been listening lately, then you know about the controversies the most reliable and biggest food chains and brands have been facing based on 'questionable' ingredients in their food items. By incorporating a paleo diet, you eat real, unprocessed food, so you know exactly where it came from, and more importantly you are in full control of what goes in your body.

## II. Nutritious

Paleo diets are rich in nutrition. Unlike most diet plans available, paleo diets are all about nutritious foods and healthy fats. This means, that you don't cut down on any important food items from your diet, but you just utilize them for better and healthier results.

## III. Stay Fit

A lot of people adapt paleo diets for weight loss purposes, which is great. Because a paleo lifestyle not only helps you lose weight, but also helps you sustain it for longer. So as long as you are on paleo, you'd stay fit. With paleo neither your metabolism suffers nor your energy levels, which means you remain active and energetic while burning your stored body fat.

People who have followed paleo diets have experienced the following benefits:

I. Improved sleep
II. Mental clarity
III. Clearer skin
IV. Healthier looking hair
V. Stable and increased energy levels
VI. Healthier gut flora
VII. Reduced allergies

VIII. Better absorption of nutrients

IX. Higher immune function

X. Muscle growth

XI. Less gas and bloating

XII. Improved glucose tolerance

Evidently, a paleo diet has many more benefits than simple weight loss. It is a complete dietary solution for all your body and health needs, and the best part is they come at almost no added cost, just healthier alternatives to your current lifestyle.

# Food items to Stock Your Pantry With

## Fats and Oils

I. Avocado oil

II. Ghee

III. Bacon fat

IV. Coconut oil

V. Macadamia oil

VI. Extra virgin olive oil

VII. Walnut oil

VIII. Sesame Oil

You don't necessarily have to stock using all the above. In the recipes below we have most commonly used bacon fat, extra virgin olive oil and coconut oil. You can alternate using whatever you prefer or is available.

## Canned and Jarred Goods

I. Olives

II. Oysters

III. Pickles

IV. Pumpkins

V. Tomato paste/sauce

VI. Tuna- wild

VII. Coconut milk

VIII.   Capers

IX.   Coconut water/juice

X.   Sweet potato

XI.   Salmon-wild

XII.   Sardines-wild

XIII.   Tahini

## *Nuts, Dried Fruits and Seeds*

I.   Almonds

II.   Banana chips

III.   Chestnuts

IV.   Coconut butter

V.   Coconut flakes/shredded

VI.   Dried apples

VII.   Dried apricots

VIII.   Pistachios

IX.   Sesame seeds

X.   Walnuts

XI.   Pecans

XII.   Hazelnuts

XIII.   Dried Raspberries

XIV.   Dried mango

XV.   Dried figs

XVI.   Dried currants

XVII.   Dates

## *Herbs and Spices*

I.   Sea salt

II.   Sage

III.   Black pepper

IV.   Cilantro

V.   Cinnamon

VI.   Cayenne

VII.    Basil

VIII.    Celery seed

IX.    Mint

X.    Nutmeg

XI.    Onion powder

XII.    Paprika

XIII.    Oregano

XIV.    Garlic

XV.    Clove

XVI.    Coriander

XVII.    Fennel Curry

XVIII.    Dill

XIX.    Turmeric

XX.    Peppercorns

XXI.    Rosemary

XXII.    Pumpkin pie spice

XXIII.    Vanilla

These are some of the most common spices used. You can of course add more based on your likings and preferences.

# Breakfast

## Pumpkin Cranberry Muffins

*Makes: 12 Muffins*

*Nutritional Info: (per muffin)*

*Calories: 174*

*Total fat 12g*

*Cholesterol: 106mg*

*Protein: 5g*

**Preparation Time: 15 minutes**

**Cooking Time: 40 Minutes**

### Ingredients:

I. 6 eggs, beaten
II. ½ cup coconut flour
III. 1 tsp vanilla
IV. ¼ cup honey or maple syrup
V. ¼ tsp baking soda
VI. ½ cup fresh cranberries
VII. 1 tbsp pumpkin pie spice
VIII. ½ cup coconut oil or butter
IX. ¼ cup pumpkin puree (remove excess water if you are using homemade)
X. ½ tsp sea salt

### Method:

1. Preheat the oven to 350F.
2. Mix together butter or oil, pumpkin, eggs, vanilla extract and honey or maple syrup in a large bowl and whisk well.

3. Add the rest of the ingredients, except cranberries and stir until combined.

4. Fold in the cranberries and scoop the batter in lined muffin cups. Use ¼ cup batter for each cup.

5. Make for 35-40 minutes.

# Vanilla Almond Sponge Bread

*Makes: 6*

## Nutritional Info: (per serving)

*Calories: 156*

*Total fat: 12g*

*Cholesterol: 222mg*

*Protein: 8g*

## Preparation Time: 5 minutes

## Cooking Time: 40 minutes

## Ingredients:

| | |
|---|---|
| I. | 2 tbsp butter |
| II. | 6 eggs |
| III. | ¼ cup coconut flour |
| IV. | 1 tsp vanilla extract |
| V. | Nutmeg cinnamon, as much as you wish to add |
| VI. | 2 tbsp coconut milk |
| VII. | ½ tsp baking soda |
| VIII. | Sliced almonds for garnishing |

## Method:

1. Preheat the oven to 350F.
2. Mix all the ingredients (except the almonds) with melted butter in a large bowl.
3. Line a 9X9 inch pan with parchment and pour the mixture in.
4. Sprinkle the almonds on top.
5. Bake for 40 minutes, usually it takes lesser time. Check with a toothpick after 30 minutes to see if it comes clean.

# Pumpkin Tahini Hot Cereal

*Makes: 4 servings*

*Nutritional Info: (per serving)*

*Calories: 92*

*Total fat: 4g*

*Cholesterol: 0mg*

*Protein: 2g*

*Preparation Time: 5 minutes*

*Cooking Time: 5 minutes*

## Ingredients:

I. 1 tbsp tahini
II. ¼ cup warm water
III. 1 tsp. cinnamon
IV. ½ cup canned pumpkin
V. 2 tbsp. raisins
VI. 2 tbsp shredded coconut
VII. 2 tbsp. honey or maple syrup
VIII. 1 tsp vanilla

## Method:

1. Add all the ingredients in a sauce pan and heat over low heat for about 5 minutes.

# Coconut Grain Free Porridge

*Makes: 2 Servings*

*Nutritional Info: (per serving)*

*Calories: 176*

*Total fat: 13g*

*Cholesterol: 0mg*

*Protein: 3g*

**Preparation Time: 5 minutes**

**Cooking Time: 5 minutes**

## Ingredients:

I.   2 tbsp almond butter
II.  ¼ tsp vanilla extract
III. ¼ cup shredded coconut
IV.  ½ tsp cinnamon
V.   6 tbsp coconut milk or warm water
VI.  1 tsp maple syrup or honey
VII. Sliced almonds for garnish

## Method:

1. Combine all the ingredients, except for the almonds in a medium bowl and mix well.
2. Add the ingredients to a small saucepan and heat it on low heat until you get the desired temperature for the porridge.
3. Transfer to the serving bowl and garnish with the almonds.

# Apple Streusel Egg Muffins

*Makes: 12 muffins*

*Nutritional Info: (per serving)*

*Calories: 111*

*Total fat: 6g*

*Cholesterol: 159mg*

*Protein: 5g*

*Preparation Time: 15 minutes*

*Cooking Time: 40 minutes*

## Ingredients:

I.   3 large apples, chopped into small pieces (you can also use peeled apples if you prefer)

II.   2 tbsp cinnamon

III.   3 tbsp warm water

IV.   1 ½ tbsp coconut oil or butter, melted

V.   3 tbsp warm water

VI.   3 tbsp coconut milk

VII.   ¼ tsp baking soda

VIII.   1 ½ tbsp coconut flour

## Method:

1. Preheat oven to 350F.
2. Sauté the apples, 1 ½ tsp of cinnamon, oil or butter and water until the apples become saucy. Allow the mixture to cool.
3. Whisk butter, eggs, coconut flour, ½ tsp of cinnamon, baking powder and salt in a mixing bowl. Add the cooled down apple mixture (You can save some of the mixture for garnishing).

4.  Spoon ¼ cup of the apple and egg picture into lined muffin cups. Add about one teaspoon of the apple mixture atop.

5.  Bake for 40 minutes. You can also replace the apples with bananas or cooked pears.

# Zucchini Pancakes

*Makes: 12 pancakes*

*Nutritional Info: (per pancake)*

*Calories: 62*

*Total fat: 3g*

*Cholesterol: 112mg*

*Protein: 4g*

**Preparation Time: 10 minutes**

**Cooking Time: 30 minutes**

## Ingredients:

I. ¼ cup coconut flour
II. ½ tsp granulated garlic
III. 6 eggs
IV. ¼ tsp sea salt
V. ¼ tsp black pepper
VI. ¼ cup bacon fat for cooking
VII. 4 cups shredded zucchini (2 large zucchinis)

## Method:

1. Sift the flour into the garlic powder, eggs, salt and pepper and beat them well.
2. Place zucchini in a nut milk bag or cheese cloth and try to squeeze some of the vegetable's water out.
3. Mix salt, pepper and shredded zucchini in the egg and flour mixture.
4. Place a cast iron skillet or enameled non-stick on medium low heat and add the bacon fat.
5. Spoon the mixture into the cakes and cook on each side for 3-4 minutes.
6. These are best served warm. You can serve separately or with bacon or sausage.

# Bacon Egg Salad

*Makes: 3 servings*

*Nutritional Info: (per serving)*

*Calories: 515*

*Total fat: 64g*

*Cholesterol: 907g*

*Protein: 37g*

*Preparation Time: 10 minutes*

*Cooking Time: 10 minutes*

## Ingredients:

I. 12 eggs, boiled and mashed
II. Sea salt and pepper to taste
III. ¼ cup Baconnaise (recipe available below)
IV. 12 slices bacon, (use the bacon drippings for the dressing)
V. Juice of 2 lemons
VI. 2 tbsp fresh chives

## Method:

1. Mix Baconnaise, eggs, sea salt, black pepper, chopped chives, chopped black peppers and bacon fat in a salad bowl. You can add some nutmegs or almonds for added texture and taste.

2. **Bacconaise Recipe:** In a medium bowl, add 2 egg yolks, 1 tbsp vinegar or egg yolks and 1 tsp Dijon mustard. Whisk until the mixture becomes bright yellow. Add ¼ cup bacon fat to the mixture and whisk well. Slowly keep on adding more bacon fat (total of ¾ cups of bacon fat) until it gets a thick and light mayo-like texture. You will get better results by using a food processor. This would get you around ¾ cups of Baconnaise. You can make a good batch and refrigerate it for future use.

# Sweet Potato Pancakes

*Makes: 5 servings*

*Nutritional Info: (per serving)*

*Calories: 124*

*Total fat: 6g*

*Cholesterol: 127 mg*

*Protein: 5g*

**Preparation Time: 10 minutes**

**Cooking Time: 10 minutes**

## Ingredients:

I.    Coconut oil, as required
II.   2 tsp coconut flour
III.  3 eggs
IV.   ¼ tsp ground ginger
V.    ½ tsp cinnamon
VI.   2 cups shredded sweet potatoes
VII.  ¼ tsp sea salt

## Method:

1. Beat the eggs and add the flour, spices and beets. Mix well until the mixture is well combined.
2. Heat an iron skillet over medium low heat and add the coconut oil, enough to coat the pan for shallow frying.
3. Spoon the mixture into the pan into small cakes. Cook on both sides for a minute each.
4. These are best served warm. You can also serve with eggs or bacon.

# Lunch

## Artichoke and Lemon Chicken

***Makes: 4 servings***

***Nutritional Info: (per serving)***

*Calories: 437*

*Total fat: 32g*

*Cholesterol: 49mg*

*Protein: 23g*

**Preparation Time: 5 minutes**

**Cooking Time: 45 minutes**

### Ingredients:

| | |
|---|---|
| I. | 1 large sweet onion, sliced |
| II. | 1 ½ lbs chicken tenders |
| III. | 1 can artichoke hearts, rinsed and drained |
| IV. | Fish sauce |
| V. | 4 tbsp ghee |
| VI. | ½ cup capers |
| VII. | Zest and juice of 2 lemons |
| VIII. | Black pepper |

### Method:

1. Preheat the oven to 375F.
2. Heat a cast iron pan and melt 1 tbsp of ghee.
3. Add capers, lemon juice, artichoke hearts, fish sauce, zest and black pepper. Sauté these ingredients for a minute.
4. Remove from heat and mix in the chicken tenders.

5. Drizzled the rest of the ghee on top and bake for 45 minutes, or until the chicken is well cooked.

# Taco Salad

**Makes: 4 servings**

**Nutritional Info: (per serving)**

*Calories: 225*

*Total fat: 13g*

*Cholesterol: 35mg*

*Protein: 15g*

**Preparation Time: 5 minutes**

**Cooking Time: 15 minutes**

## Ingredients:

I. 1lb ground beef
II. 2 tbsp All natural taco mix
III. 1 large tomato, chopped
IV. 1 head ice berg lettuce, shredded or torn
V. 1 avocado, chopped
VI. Salt to taste
VII. 1 cup bell peppers, chopped

## Method:

1. Brown the ground beef in a frying pan.
2. Drain the fat and add ½ cup water and the taco mix and boil over low heat for 10 minutes.
3. Toss the vegetables in a salad bowl and add the beef. This taco free alternative is both delicious and filling. You can add nuts of your choice for extra crunch.

# Duck with Cherry Sauce

*Makes: 2 servings*

*Nutritional Info: (per serving)*

*Calories: 236*

*Total fat: 11g*

*Cholesterol: 105mg*

*Protein: 25g*

**Preparation Time: 10 minutes**

**Cooking Time: 60-80 minutes**

## Ingredients:

I.    2 duck breasts or legs
II.   ¼ tsp dry sage
III.  ¼ tsp dried rosemary
IV.   ¾ cup fresh, frozen or dried cherries (if using dried then soak in warm water for about an hour)
V.    ½ tsp sea salt
VI.   A sprig of fresh rosemary

## Method:

1. Preheat the oven to 320F.
2. Add the spices to the duck and place it in a roasting pan or oven safe skillet.
3. Roast the duck until it is brown and crispy, approx 60-80 minutes.
4. Simmer the cherries with rosemary and water until the cherries begin to break.
5. Remove the rosemary and mash the fruit into a chunky sauce.
6. Add the sauce to the duck while serving. You can save the duck fat for salads or roasting root vegetables.

# Simple Shrimp Ceviche

*Makes: 4 servings*

*Nutritional Info: (per serving)*

*Calories: 228*

*Total fat: 7g*

*Cholesterol: 161mg*

*Protein: 24g*

**Preparation Time: 10 minutes**

**Cooking Time: 4 minutes**

## Ingredients:

I.  ½ cucumber
II.  ½ red bell pepper
III.  ½ jicama bulb
IV.  1 avocado
V.  2-3 garlic cloves
VI.  1 small shallot
VII.  1 lb cooked, peeled and deveined shrimp
VIII.  Sea salt and pepper to taste
IX.  Juice of 1 lime
X.  Handful of fresh cilantro
XI.  Juice of 2 lemons

## Method:

1. Finely dice the cucumber, jicama, shallot, garlic and pepper and add in a large mixing bowl. Slit open and dice the avocado and add to the bowl along with chopped cilantro.
2. Chop the shrimp into small bites and mix it with the rest of the ingredients.

3. Chill the mixture for about 30 minutes before serving. Add sea salt and pepper before serving.

4. You can also add mango or pineapple chunks for the added flavor.

# Baked Beets with Fennel

*Makes: 3-4 servings*

*Nutritional Info: (per serving)*

*Calories: 204*

*Total fat: 14g*

*Cholesterol: 0mg*

*Protein: 3g*

*Preparation Time: 10 minutes*

*Cooking Time: 45-50 minutes*

## Ingredients:

I. 2 large beets, peeled and cut into 1 inch cubes
II. ½ orange, peeled and sliced into ½ inch pieces
III. 2 tbsp coconut oil or butter
IV. 1 fennel bulb, sliced into ¼ inch strips
V. Sea salt and freshly ground pepper to taste

## Method:

1. Preheat the oven to 375F.
2. Add all the ingredients in a mixing bowl.
3. Melt the oil or butter and pour over the mixture. Toss the mixture until it is well coated with the butter or oil.
4. Spread the mixture in a lined baking tray and season with sea salt and pepper. Bake until the beets are fork-tender, around 45-50 minutes.

# Seared Lamb Chops with Rosemary Salt

*Makes: 4 servings*

*Nutritional Info: (per serving)*

*Calories: 400*

*Total fat: 31g*

*Cholesterol: 104mg*

*Protein: 30g*

**Preparation Time:10 minutes**

**Cooking Time: 5 minutes**

## Ingredients:

I.    8 lamb rib chops
II.   1 tbsp bacon fat or coconut oil
III.  2 tbsp dried, ground rosemary
IV.   ¼ tsp coarse sea salt

## Method:

1. Preheat the oven to 400F.
2. Heat a large oven safe stainless steel or cast iron skillet on medium heat and add the bacon fat.
3. Season the lamb chops with rosemary, salt and pepper.
4. Sear each side of the chop for about 2 minutes and then place the pan in the oven for another 2 minutes.

# Grain Free Salmon Cakes

*Makes: 2 servings*

*Nutritional Info: (per serving)*

*Calories: 186*

*Total fat: 8g*

*Cholesterol: 152mg*

*Protein: 21g*

*Preparation Time: 10 minutes*

*Cooking Time: 15 minutes*

## Ingredients:

I.    6 oz cooked wild salmon, mashed up
II.   ¼ red onion, finely chopped
III.  1 large clove of garlic, finely chopped or pressed
IV.   1-2 tbsp finely chopped chives
V.    1 egg
VI.   1 tsp Dijon mustard
VII.  Sea salt and pepper to taste
VIII. 1 tsp coconut flour
IX.   Zest and juice of ½ lemon
X.    Coconut oil, as required for shallow frying

## Method:

1. Combine garlic, onion, mustard, chives, egg, pepper, coconut flour and sea salt in a mixing bowl.
2. Add the salmon and mix well. Make small patties.
3. Heat a small iron skillet with the desired amount of oil. Cook the patties for about 2-3 minutes on each side or until well browned.

4. You can garnish the patties with onions, chives, lemon juice and lemon zest while serving. You can serve these with salad greens.

5. This recipe can also be made from other leftover fish, tuna or crab meat.

# Bacon Wrapped Smoky Chicken Thighs

*Makes: 4 Servings*

*Nutritional Info: (per serving)*

*Calories:  195*

*Total fat: 12g*

*Cholesterol: 67mg*

*Protein: 19g*

**Preparation Time: 10 minutes**

**Cooking Time: 40 minutes**

## Ingredients:

I. 4 bone-in skinless chicken thighs
II. 2 tsp smoky spice blend
III. 8 slices bacon

**(Recipe for Smokey Spice Blend:** Add 1 tbsp each of chipotle powder, smoked paprika, sea salt and onion powder and ½ tbsp each of cinnamon and black pepper. Store the rest for future use.)

## Method:

1. Preheat the oven to 375F.
2. Sprinkle the chicken thighs with 1 tsp of the mixed spice.
3. Wrap each chicken thigh with 2 strips of bacon.
4. Sprinkle the remaining spice blend on top and bake for approx 40 minutes.

# Grain Free Sausage and Apple Dressing

*Makes: 6 servings*

*Nutritional Info: (per serving)*

*Calories: 336*

*Total fat: 22g*

*Cholesterol: 58mg*

*Protein: 14g*

*Preparation Time: 15 minutes*

*Cooking Time: 30 minutes*

## Ingredients:

I. 1 lb ground sausage meat, (you can make your own too by adding 1 tbsp of onion powder, garlic powder, paprika, ground fennel seed and 1tsp of sea salt, ground pepper, a dash of cayenne and 3-4 leaves of chopped fresh sage to 1lb of your preferred ground meat (pork or chicken)

II. 1 tbsp butter or bacon fat

III. 3 stalks of celery, chopped into small pieces

IV. 1 onion, chopped into small pieces

V. 2 green apples, chopped into small pieces

VI. Sea salt and pepper to taste

VII. 1 cup roasted chestnuts, roughly chopped

VIII. 4-6 fresh sage leaves

IX. ¼ cup dried or fresh cranberries

X. ¼ cup chicken or turkey stock

## Method:

1. Brown the sausage on medium low heat.

2. Sauté the celery, onion, apples and seasoning in bacon or sausage fat.

3. Add the roasted chestnuts, stock and cranberries in a pan and simmer over medium low heat for 2-3 minutes.

4. Combine all the mixtures and serve. You can also brown the mixture together a bit before serving.

# Spinach Salad with Orange and Fresh Mint Vinaigrette

*Makes: 2 servings*

*Nutritional Info: (per serving)*

*Calories: 170*

*Total fat: 14g*

*Cholesterol: 0mg*

*Protein: 3g*

**Preparation Time: 10 minutes**

**Cooking Time: 0 minutes**

## Ingredients:

I.   4 cups baby spinach
II.  1 small zucchini, raw and shredded
III. 1 small red beet, peeled and shredded

### For the Vinaigrette:

I.    Zest and juice of 1 orange or lemon
II.   1 tbsp raw apple cider vinegar
III.  ½ tsp Dijon mustard
IV.   2 tbsp melted coconut oil or bacon fat
V.    4 fresh spearmint leaves, finely chopped
VI.   Sea salt and pepper to taste
VII.  Pinch of garlic powder or grated fresh garlic

## Method:

1. Add the shredded beet, zucchini and spinach in a salad bowl.
2. Whisk the dressing ingredients together and toss them in the salad.

3. You can garnish with sprig of mint and orange slices.

4. You can also add steak, chicken or fish.

# Turkey and Bacon Salad

*Makes: 1 serving*

*Nutritional Info: (per serving)*

*Calories: 561*

*Total fat: 34g*

*Cholesterol: 100mg*

*Protein: 45g*

**Preparation Time: 10 minutes**

**Cooking Time: 30 minutes**

## Ingredients:

I. 2 cups mixed baby lettuces
II. 2 slices bacon
III. ¼ of avocado, cut into chunks
IV. 4 oz roasted turkey
V. 2 tbsp Thinly sliced red onion
VI. 1 tbsp extra virgin olive oil
VII. 1 tbsp fresh chives, chopped
VIII. Juice of ½ lemon

## Method:

1. Bake the bacon at 375F for around 30 minutes. You can also pan fry it.
2. Layer the ingredients over the greens and top with lemon and olive oil. Add sea salt and black pepper to taste.

# Rosemary Lemon Broiled Salmon

*Makes: 3-4 servings*

*Nutritional Info: (per serving)*

*Calories: 239*

*Total fat: 13g*

*Cholesterol: 88mg*

*Protein: 28g*

**Preparation Time: 10 minutes**

**Cooking Time: 15 minutes**

## Ingredients:

I.   1 lb salmon
II.  1 tsp rosemary salt blend (made with adding dried rosemary and coarse sea salt)
III. 2 tbsp butter or coconut oil

## Method:

1. Preheat the oven to low broil setting.
2. Add the butter or oil to a baking dish and place salmon on top.
3. Sprinkle with rosemary salt and add some more butter or oil on top. Add slices of lemon on top.
4. Broil for about 10-15 minutes or until the salmon is cooked properly.

# Snacks

## Kale Chips

*Makes: 2-3 servings*

*Nutritional Info: (per serving)*

Calories: 47

Total fat: 4g

Cholesterol: 0mg

Protein: 1g

**Preparation Time: 5 minutes**

**Cooking Time: 15 minutes**

### Ingredients:

I.     1 large bunch of kale, remove the stems and roughly chop the leaves
II.    Sea salt to taste
III.   1-2 tbsp coconut oil, melted
IV.    Garlic powder, as desired

### Method:

1. Preheat the oven to 359 degrees.
2. Place the kale on a baking sheet and drizzle with oil. Use your hands to blend the oil well. There should be enough to lightly coat the leaves rather than drench them with oil.
3. Sprinkle with sea salt and garlic powder.
4. Bake for 10-15 minutes or until the kale edges become brown.
5. Let the leaves be in the oven until they become crispy.  You can also cool them off on the countertop.
6. You can add sesame seeds, chili powder,  raw cheese etc. for added flavor.

# Chicken Liver Pate

*Makes: 4 servings*

*Nutritional Info: (per serving)*

*Calories: 346*

*Total fat: 29g*

*Cholesterol: 447mg*

*Protein: 20g*

*Preparation Time: 10 minutes*

*Cooking Time: 10 minutes*

## Ingredients:

I.    1lb chicken liver, you can also use other livers if you like
II.   ½ cup balsamic vinegar
III.  1 small onion, chopped
IV.   2-4 garlic cloves, crush
V.    1 sprig fresh rosemary
VI.   1tsp Dijon mustard
VII.  2 sprigs fresh thyme
VIII. ½ cup butter or coconut oil
IX.   1 tbsp fresh lemon juice
X.    1 tbsp cracked black pepper
XI.   Sea salt to taste

## Method:

1. Sauté the onions and liver in butter until the onions are tender and the liver is browned.
2. Add vinegar, mustard, garlic, lemon juice and herbs to the liver and cook until the liquid is almost gone.

3. Blend the mixture in the food processor until it becomes a smooth paste. Add 1 tbsp of butter for added creamy consistency.

4. Refrigerate the pate before serving

5. You can enjoy this with cucumber, pepper, celery or carrot sticks.

# Mango Salsa

*Makes: 4 servings*

*Nutritional Info: (per serving)*

*Calories: 144*

*Total fat: 7g*

*Cholesterol: 0mg*

*Protein: 1g*

**Preparation Time:5 minutes**

**Cooking Time: 0 minutes**

## Ingredients:

I. 1 small red bell pepper, finely diced
II. 2 large mangoes, diced
III. 1 jalapeno pepper, finely diced
IV. 2-4 tbsp of diced fresh cilantro
V. 1 large shallot, finely diced
VI. 1 clove of garlic, pressed
VII. 1 lime juice
VIII. Sea salt and pepper to taste
IX. 2 tbsp extra virgin olive oil

## Method:

1. Combine all the ingredients and chill before serving. You can also substitute mangoes with peaches, tomatoes or pineapples.

# Quick Guacamole Recipe

*Makes: 2 servings*

*Nutritional Info: (per serving)*

*Calories: 126*

*Total fat: 11g*

*Cholesterol: 0mg*

*Protein: 2g*

**Preparation Time: 5 minutes**

**Cooking Time: 0 minutes**

## Ingredients:

I.  1 avocado, cubed or mashed
II. 1 tbsp shallot, diced
III. ½ lime juice
IV. Fresh cilantro, as required
V.  Sea salt and black pepper to taste

## Method:

1. Mix all the ingredients together for a quick snack or you can serve them with fish, beef, pork or chicken for a complete meal.

# Fulfilling Green Juice

*Makes: 1 serving*

*Nutritional Info: (per serving)*

*Calories: 145*

*Total fat: 1g*

*Cholesterol: 0mg*

*Protein: 6g*

*Preparation Time: 5 minutes*

*Cooking Time: 0 minutes*

## Ingredients:

I.   3-4 stalks of celery
II.  ½ of a cucumber
III. 4 stems of kale
IV.  ½ green apple
V.   2-3 broccoli stems
VI.  ½ lemon

## Method:

1. Blend the ingredients together in a blender until smooth. You might need to add water to set the right smoothness. You can alter the quantity of the ingredients to better suit your liking.

# Candied Carrots

*Makes: 4 servings*

*Nutritional Info: (per serving)*

*Calories: 137*

*Total fat: 7g*

*Cholesterol: 19g*

*Protein: 2g*

**Preparation Time: 5 minutes**

**Cooking Time: 30 minutes**

## Ingredients:

I.    8 large carrots, peeled and chopped into small pieces
II.   2 tbsp melted coconut oil
III.  Sea salt to taste
IV.   4 dates, pitted and chopped

## Method:

1. Preheat the oven to 375F.
2. Place the dates and carrots in an oven safe dish and drizzled with coconut oil.
3. Toss to coat the carrots and dates with the oil. Sprinkle with sea salt to taste.
4. Bake until the carrots are fork tender, about 20-30 minutes.

# Dinner

## Thanksgiving Meatballs

*Makes: 24 meatballs approx.*

*Nutritional Info: (per serving)*

*Calories: 282*

*Total fat: 21g*

*Cholesterol: 54mg*

*Protein: 14g*

**Preparation Time: 20 minutes**

**Cooking Time: 25-30 minutes**

### Ingredients:

I. 2 lb ground pork
II. 2 tsp butter, coconut oil or bacon fat
III. 2 tbsp Italian Sausage Spice Blend
IV. ¼ cup onion, finely chopped
V. ¼ cup carrot, grated
VI. ¼ cup celery, finely chopped
VII. ¼ cup chestnuts, finely chopped (use can also use pecans or walnuts)

### Method:

1. Preheat the oven to 425F.
2. Combine the spice blend and pork in a medium bowl until it is well seasoned.
3. Melt the butter/fat/oil on a skillet on medium heat. Add the celery, onions and carrots to the pan and sauté until the celery and onions become translucent. Add the nuts and cook for another 2 minutes.
4. Set the mixture aside to cool down.

5. Combine the mixture with ground pork and make them into 24 meatballs.

6. Place the meatballs on a baking sheet or oven safe dish and cook for about 25-30 minutes.

# Spaghetti Squash Bolognese

*Makes: 4 servings*

*Nutritional Info: (per serving)*

*Calories: 370*

*Total fat: 25g*

*Cholesterol: 55mg*

*Protein: 15g*

*Preparation Time: 15 minutes*

*Cooking Time: 60 minutes*

## Ingredients:

I. 1 spaghetti squash
II. 2 tbsp bacon fat
III. 1 carrot, finely chopped
IV. 1 onion, finely diced
V. 1 stalk of celery, finely diced
VI. 1 clove of garlic, grated
VII. ½ lb ground pork
VIII. ½ lb beef or veal
IX. 4 slices bacon, chopped
X. 3 ounces tomato paste
XI. ½ cup coconut milk
XII. Sea salt and black pepper to taste
XIII. ½ cup coconut milk

## Method:

1. Preheat the oven to 375F.
2. Slice the spaghetti squash in half and scoop out the seeds. Sprinkle with sea salt and pepper.

3. Place both spaghetti squash halves face down on an oven safe dish or baking sheet. Roast for about 35-40 minutes, or until the flesh becomes translucent.

4. Cool down the squash and then scoop the flesh out and into a serving bowl.

5. Melt the bacon fat over a medium high heat and sauté the carrots, onions and celery until the onions and celery become translucent. Add the garlic and cook for another minute.

6. Add the bacon, veal and pork and cook until all the ingredients are browned. Add tomato paste and coconut milk to the proteins and simmer on medium low heat for about 30 minutes. Add pepper and sea salt to taste.

7. Serve over the spaghetti squash.

# Supper Kebabs

*Makes: 3 servings*

*Nutritional Info: (per serving)*

*Calories: 191*

*Total fat: 4g*

*Cholesterol: 78mg*

*Protein: 34g*

**Preparation Time: 10 minutes**

**Cooking Time: 15 minutes**

## Ingredients:

I. 1 lb meat cut into 2 inch chunks
II. 2 tomatoes, cut into large chunks
III. 1 red onion, cut into large chunks
IV. Sea salt and black pepper to taste
V. Ground garlic powder to taste
VI. Oregano or rosemary to taste

## Method:

1. Sprinkle the meat with seasonings.
2. Add the vegetables and meat on skewers. Make sure you soak the wooden skewers in water before putting on the ingredients.
3. Place the skewers on a grill pan on medium high heat.
4. Cook each side for a few minutes or until browned. You can also make meat only and vegetable only skewers if you don't like your vegetables completely browned.
5. You can also add more vegetables if you like.
6. You can use shrimps, pork, lamb, chicken or beef.

# Stuffed Bell Peppers

*Makes: 4 servings*

## Nutritional Info: (per serving)

*Calories: 296*

*Total fat: 18g*

*Cholesterol: 73mg*

*Protein: 24g*

## Preparation Time: 10 minutes

## Cooking Time: 20 minutes

## Ingredients:

- I. 1 lb ground beef/turkey
- II. 2 bell peppers
- III. 1 tbsp bacon grease or coconut oil
- IV. 4 cloves garlic, pressed
- V. ½ onion, diced
- VI. 4 small tomatoes, diced
- VII. 6 fresh basil leaves, finely chopped
- VIII. Sea salt and black pepper to taste
- IX. 2 cup baby spinach, finely chopped

## Method:

1. Preheat the oven to 375F.
2. Halve the bell peppers and roast them in the oven for 10-15 minutes.
3. Add bacon grease or oil in a large pot or sauté pan. Cook the onions over medium high until they are translucent. Add sea salt and pepper.
4. Add the garlic and tomatoes and cook for another few minutes.
5. Add the meat and break it up to make sure it is cooked through properly.

6. When the meat is cooked, add more salt and pepper if needed. Add the spinach and basil and cook for another 30 seconds.

7. Stuff the mixture in the bell peppers and serve. You can also cook the mixture in the oven for an added 10 minutes to get extra flavor.

8. You can make these in a big batch and freeze for later.

# Braised Beef Shanks

*Makes: 3 Servings*

*Nutritional Info: (per serving)*

*Calories: 414*

*Total fat: 11g*

*Cholesterol: 145mg*

*Protein: 51g*

**Preparation Time: 10 minutes**

**Cooking Time: 4-6 hours**

## Ingredients:

I. 2 large beef shanks
II. 2 tbsp apple cider vinegar or balsamic vinegar
III. 4 cloves garlic
IV. 1-2 sprigs fresh rosemary
V. Sea salt and black pepper to taste
VI. 2-3 cups chicken stock or homemade broth

## Method:

1. Add all the ingredients in a crock pot and cook for about 4-6 hours or until the meat easily falls apart using a fork.
2. You can garnish with sautéed kales using coconut oil and onion powder.

# Grilled Garden Salad

*Makes: 1 serving*

*Nutritional Info: (per serving)*

*Calories: 238*

*Total fat: 16g*

*Cholesterol: 25mg*

*Protein: 10g*

*Preparation Time: 5 minutes*

*Cooking Time: 10 minutes*

## Ingredients:

I. 6-8oz grilled chicken
II. 2 cups mixed greens, rinsed and dried
III. 1 small tomato, sliced
IV. 1 small red onion, sliced and sautéed or grilled
V. ½ small bell pepper, sliced

### For the Dressing:

1 tbsp fresh lemon juice

Sea salt and black pepper to taste

1 tbsp extra virgin olive oil

## Method:

1. Mix the ingredients for the dressing well.
2. Add all the vegetables and the chicken in a salad bowl and top with the dressing.

# Stuffed Mushrooms

*Makes: 3 Servings*

*Nutritional Info: (per serving)*

*Calories: 335*

*Total fat: 26g*

*Cholesterol: 63mg*

*Protein: 18g*

**Preparation Time: 10 minutes**

**Cooking Time: 60 minutes**

## Ingredients:

I. 4 large Portobello mushroom caps
II. ½ red bell pepper, minced
III. ½ onion, mined
IV. 1 tbsp bacon fat
V. 1lb ground pork
VI. 1 clove garlic, pressed
VII. 2 cups spinach, finely chopped
VIII. 1 tsp fennel seeds, crushed
IX. ½ tsp garlic powder, ground sage and onion powder each
X. 1 tsp dried parsley

## Method:

1. Preheat the oven to 450F.
2. Bake the mushrooms for about 10 minutes with cap side down.
3. Heat the bacon fat in a large skillet over medium heat.
4. Add pepper and onions and sauté for 3 minutes. Add the pork and the spices to the pan and cook until the pork is cooked.
5. Add the garlic and spinach.

6. Spoon the mixture in the mushroom caps and cook for another 15-20 minutes or until the stuffing is browned.

# Asian Turkey Burgers

*Makes: 4 servings*

*Nutritional Info: (per serving)*

*Calories:  194*

*Total fat: 11g*

*Cholesterol: 84mg*

*Protein: 23g*

**Preparation Time: 5 minutes**

**Cooking Time: 15 minutes**

## Ingredients:

I.    1 lb ground turkey
II.   Sprigs of fresh cilantro
III.  1 tbsp Indian Spice Blend

Indian Spice Blend Recipe*: Add 2 tbsp of onion powder, 2 tsp curry powder, 2 tsp coriander,1/2 tsp red flakes, 1 tsp sea salt and black pepper, ½ tsp cinnamon. This should make about 5 tbsp of Indian Spice Blend. You can make a good batch to add to your spice mixes.*

## Method:

1. Combine the turkey with the spice mix until well mixed. Form four patties out of the mixture.
2. You can choose to either cook on skillet or grill the patties over medium high heat. Cook for about 4 minutes on each side.
3. You can use Portobello mushrooms as buns and grill for an added 10 minutes inside the 'buns'. You can also serve the patties with a fresh salad.

# Squash Fettuccine with Pesto Shrimps

*Makes: 2 servings*

*Nutritional Info: (per serving)*

*Calories:  410*

*Total fat: 41g*

*Cholesterol: 65mg*

*Protein: 10g*

*Preparation Time:10 minutes*

*Cooking Time: 10 minutes*

## Ingredients:

   I.    2 dozen large shrimps

   II.   Sea salt and pepper to taste

   III.  4 yellow squash or zucchini

### For the Pesto:

   I.    1 bunch cilantro, rinsed and dried

   II.   ½ cup macadamia nuts

   III.  1 clove garlic

   IV.  Sea salt and pepper to taste

   V.   ½ cup extra virgin olive oil

## Method:

1. Combine all the pesto ingredients and blend them in a food processor until smooth.
2. Peel and devein the shrimps.
3. Boil about an inch of water in a large sauce pan with a steamer basket in the middle.

4. Julienne or peel the squash until the seedy part and add to the steamer. Steam the squash noodles for about 5 minutes.

5. Steam the shrimps after the squash noodles for 3 minutes or until they are pink.

6. Toss the pesto, squash noodles and shrimps in a bowl and serve.

# Roasted Winter Squash

**Makes: 2 Servings**

**Nutritional Info: (per serving)**

*Calories: 144*

*Total fat: 14g*

*Cholesterol: 0mg*

*Protein: 1g*

**Preparation Time: 10 minutes**

**Cooking Time: 30-60 minutes**

## Ingredients:

I.   1 winter squash, cut in half with seeds scooped out and disposed
II.  Cinnamon to taste
III. 2 tbsp coconut cream or coconut butter
IV.  Sea salt to taste

## Method:

1. Preheat the oven to 375F.
2. Place both the halves of squash on a roasting dish or pan and cook until the squash becomes soft. This could anywhere between 20-60 minutes depending on the size.
3. Remove from the oven and top it with sea salt and coconut butter.

# Tomato and Avocado Salad

*Makes: 1 serving*

*Nutritional Info: (per serving)*

*Calories: 287*

*Total fat: 25g*

*Cholesterol: 0mg*

*Protein: 4g*

**Preparation Time: 5 minutes**

**Cooking Time: 0 minutes**

## Ingredients:

I. ½ avocado, diced into small pieces
II. 2 Early Girl tomatoes, cut into wedges
III. 1 wedge of lemon
IV. Extra Virgin Olive Oil, according to taste
V. 1 sprig of cilantro, chopped
VI. Sea salt to taste

## Method:

1. Combine avocado, tomatoes and cilantro in a salad bowl.
2. Drizzle olive oil and squeeze lemon on top. Add sea salt and toss the ingredients.
3. You can also use basil if cilantro isn't available. You can also add grilled chicken or fish to make it more filling.

# Baked Chicken Legs

*Makes: 2 servings*

*Nutritional Info: (per serving)*

*Calories: 124*

*Total fat: 9g*

*Cholesterol: 42mg*

*Protein: 9g*

**Preparation Time: 5 minutes**

**Cooking Time: 15 minutes**

## Ingredients:

I.     2 whole chicken legs
II.    Sea salt to taste
III.   Black pepper to taste
IV.   1 tbsp dried or fresh rosemary
V.    ½ tsp garlic powder
VI.   Coconut oil as much required
VII.  1 tsp paprika

## Method:

1. Preheat the oven to 375F.
2. Dry the chicken legs with kitchen towel and brush with coconut oil.
3. Sprinkle the legs with the spices. You can add less or more depending on your preferences.
4. Bake the legs in a shallow baking dish for 5-10 minutes. Open the oven door and baste the chicken drippings back on top.
5. Bake until the chicken is properly cooked.
6. You can add or replace with other spices like onion powder, sage etc.

# Kale and Carrot Salad with Tahini Dressing

*Makes: 2 Servings*

*Nutritional Info: (per serving)*

*Calories: 100*

*Total fat: 4g*

*Cholesterol: 0mg*

*Protein: 4g*

*Preparation Time: 5 minutes*

*Cooking Time: 0 minutes*

## Ingredients:

I. 1-2 tbsp tahini
II. 1 carrot, chopped into small pieces
III. 1 bunch kale
IV. 1 tbsp apple cider vinegar
V. 1 tsp lemon juice
VI. 1 tbsp rice wine vinegar
VII. 1 clove of garlic, pressed
VIII. Sea salt and pepper to taste
IX. 1 tsp raw honey

## Method:

1. Remove kale from stalks and roughly chop them. Squeeze the kale in your hands to make them more soft and easy to chew.
2. Add kale to the carrots.
3. Mix lemon juice, honey, salt, pepper, apple cider, rice vinegar and lemon juice in a small bowl.
4. Pour the dressing over the salad and enjoy.
5. You can also make this salad with shredded apples, zucchini, avocado etc.

# Desserts

## Apple and Walnut Delight

*Makes: 6 servings*

*Nutritional Info: (per serving)*

*Calories:  190*

*Total fat: 13g*

*Cholesterol: 17mg*

*Protein: 3g*

**Preparation Time: 10 minutes**

**Cooking Time: 40 minutes**

### Ingredients:

I.    4 green apples
II.   ¼ cup walnuts, chopped
III.  1 cup almond meal
IV.   ¼ cup coconut oil
V.    ¼ tsp cinnamon
VI.   Sea salt as desired

### Method:

1. Preheat the oven to 375F.
2. Cut the apples into thin slices and place them equally in a baking dish.
3. Squeeze lemon juice on top.
4. Mix the rest of the ingredients in a small bowl.
5. Pour over the apples and bake for 40 minutes.

# Butter cups with Chocolate and Almonds

*Makes: 12 servings*

*Nutritional Info: (per serving)*

*Calories: 123*

*Total fat: 12g*

*Cholesterol: 0mg*

*Protein: 2g*

*Preparation Time: 15 minutes*

*Cooking Time: 0 minutes*

## Ingredients:

I. ¼ cup coconut cream concentrate
II. 1 tbsp coconut oil
III. ½ twp vanilla extract
IV. 3 tbsp almond meal
V. Dash of cinnamon
VI. Pinch of Celtic sea salt
VII. 2 tbsp almond butter
VIII. 3 tbsp unsweetened cocoa powder
IX. 3 tbsp maple syrup, divided

## Method:

1. Melt the coconut oil and add half of the coconut cream, tbsp maple syrup and vanilla extract. Blend them until they are combined.
2. Add the rest of the coconut cream and blend.
3. Whisk cocoa powder, cinnamon and almond meal into the mixture.
4. Pour the mixture into a mini muffin tin lined with paper. Only add enough to coat the bottom of each hole.
5. Place the tin in the freezer and let it freeze.

6. Whisk almond butter with a pinch of sea salt and 1 tbsp maple syrup.

7. Once the mixture is frozen, pipe the almond butter mixture using a piping bag.

# Blueberry Crumble

*Makes: 8 Servings*

## *Nutritional Info: (per serving)*

*Calories: 197*

*Total fat: 14g*

*Cholesterol: 20mg*

*Protein: 2g*

## *Preparation Time: 15 minutes*

## *Cooking Time: 30-40 minutes*

## Ingredients:

   I.    2 pints of fresh blueberries
   II.   1 cup almond flour/almond meal
   III.  Juice of 1 lemon
   IV.   ¼ cup macadamia nuts, chopped
   V.    2 tbsp maple syrup
   VI.   ¼ cup melted butter
   VII.  ¼ tsp cinnamon
   VIII. 2 pinches sea salt

## Method:

1. Preheat the oven to 375F.
2. Place the blueberries in a baking dish and squeeze half lemon over them.
3. Toss the blueberries to coat the lemon juice.
4. Combine the macadamia nuts. Almond flour, melted butter, maple syrup, cinnamon, salt and the remaining lemon juice in a small bowl and spread it over the blueberries.
5. Bake it for 30 minutes or until the blueberries are cooked and the topping is brown.

# 7 Layer Cookie Bars

*Makes: 12 Servings*

*Nutritional Info: (per serving)*

*Calories: 272*

*Total fat: 23g*

*Cholesterol: 38mg*

*Protein: 6g*

*Preparation Time: 15 minutes*

*Cooking Time: 30 minutes*

## Ingredients:

I. 13.5oz can full fat coconut milk
II. ¼ tsp vanilla extract
III. 1 tsp honey
IV. 2 large eggs
V. 2 tbsp butter
VI. 1 cup nuts, finely ground (pecans, almonds, hazelnuts)
VII. ¾ cup peanut butter chips
VIII. ¾ cup chocolate chips
IX. 1 cup shredded coconut, divided
X. ½ cup chopped walnuts

## Method:

1. Preheat the oven to 350F.
2. In a small saucepan add coconut milk, vanilla and honey and simmer over medium heat until the mixture is reduced to half, about 20 minutes. Whisk the mixture regularly to retain the smooth texture.

3. Beat the egg whites and add the almond meal and melted butter. Pour this mixture in a 9X9 pan lined with parchment paper. Spread the mixture until it is even.

4. Add layers of coconut, chocolate chips, walnuts and peanut butter chips.

5. Drizzle the coconut milk mixture on the top and sprinkle with coconut.

6. Bake for 30 minutes and then cut into mini bites or bars when cool.

# Walnut and Chocolate Truffles

*Makes: 6 servings*

*Nutritional Info: (per serving)*

*Calories: 246*

*Total fat: 22g*

*Cholesterol: 0mg*

*Protein: 4g*

*Preparation Time: 15 minutes*

*Cooking Time: 5 minutes*

## Ingredients:

I.    1 cup raw walnuts
II.   ¼ cup extra virgin coconut oil, melted
III.  ¼ cup cocoa powder, and more for rolling the truffles
IV.   Dash of sea salt
V.    3 tbsp honey

## Method:

1. Whisk in honey and cocoa powder in the melted coconut oil.
2. Finely grind the walnuts in a food processor. The walnuts should have pasty texture.
3. Combine walnuts paste with the coconut oil mixture in a mixing bowl and place it in the freezer until it sets and the coconut oil is hardened again.
4. Make balls using your hands from the mixture and roll in cocoa powder.
5. Refrigerate or freeze based on your preference.

# Chocolate Mousse

*Makes: 2 servings*

*Nutritional Info: (per serving)*

*Calories: 346*

*Total fat: 26g*

*Cholesterol:0mg*

*Protein: 6g*

*Preparation Time: 10 minutes*

*Cooking Time: 0 minutes*

## Ingredients:

| I. | 2 ripe bananas |
| II. | 2 ripe avocados |
| III. | ½ cup coconut milk |
| IV. | ½ cup unsweetened cacao powder |
| V. | ½ tsp vanilla extract |
| VI. | Pinch of sea salt |
| VII. | Pinch of cinnamon |
| VIII. | 1-2 tbsp maple syrup |
| IX. | 1 tbsp cacao nibs or 100% dark chocolate, for garnish |

## Method:

1. Scoop out the flesh of avocados and peel the bananas.
2. Add all the listed ingredients, except for garnish, in the food processor and process until well blended.
3. Serve in bowls and garnish with dark chocolate, coconut or toasted hazelnuts.

# Pumpkin Pie without Crust

**Makes: 4-6 servings**

**Nutritional Info: (per serving)**

Calories: 226

Total fat: 15g

Cholesterol: 21g

Protein: 5g

**Preparation Time: 10 minutes**

**Cooking Time: 1 hour**

## Ingredients:

I. 1 cup canned pumpkin puree
II. ¼ tsp ground ginger
III. 1 tsp cinnamon
IV. Pinch of sea salt
V. 2 eggs
VI. 2 pinches of grated nutmeg
VII. ¼ cup maple syrup
VIII. 1 cup full fat coconut milk
IX. 1 tsp vanilla extract

## Method:

1. Preheat the oven to 350F.
2. Boil a pot of water, with enough water to fill the baking pan.
3. Combine all the spices and the pumpkin puree in a mixing bowl.
4. In another bowl, beat the eggs and add the vanilla, maple syrup and coconut milk.
5. Blend the two mixtures together until well combined.

6.  Pour the custard in ½ cup ramekins and place them in a baking pan. Add enough water to the baking pan to reach 2" high around the ramekins.
7.  Place the baking pan in the oven and bake for 60 minutes.
8.  Chill before serving.

# Sweet and Sour Gelatin Munchies

*Makes: 4 servings*

*Nutritional Info: (per serving)*

*Calories: 324*

*Total fat: 0g*

*Cholesterol: 0mg*

*Protein: 7g*

**Preparation Time: 10 minutes**

**Cooking Time: 5 minutes**

## Ingredients:

I.   ¾ cup freshly squeezed lemon juice
II.  ¼ cup water
III. ¼ cup freshly squeezed lime juice
IV.  Lemon and lime zests as desired
V.   1 tbsp maple syrup
VI.  4-5 tbsp grass fed gelatin (orange or red package)

## Method:

1. Whisk the lime juice, lemon juice, water, maple syrup, zest and gelatin together in a pot over medium-low heat until the gelatin is dissolved and the mixture becomes slurry.
2. Use a small ceramic or glass dish, it should be small enough to yield at least ½ to 1 inch thick cubes, if you would like thinner gummies to cut into worms or other shapes, use a larger pan.
3. Pour the mixture in the dish and refrigerate it for about 30 minutes or until it is completely set.

4. You can also make these with blueberries; simply replace the lemon juice with 1 cup of frozen or fresh blueberries. Just blend the mixture before adding it to the pot.

# Pumpkin Soufflé

*Makes: 4 servings*

*Nutritional Info: (per serving)*

*Calories: 216*

*Total fat: 14g*

*Cholesterol: 86mg*

*Protein: 5g*

**Preparation Time: 15 minutes**

**Cooking Time: 25-35 minutes**

## Ingredients:

I. 1 cup pumpkin
II. 4 eggs
III. 2 tbsp almond butter
IV. ¼ cup coconut oil
V. 6 tbsp maple syrup
VI. ¼ tsp baking soda
VII. 1 tsp pumpkin pie spice
VIII. 1 tbsp coconut flour
IX. Pinch of sea salt

## Method:

1. Preheat the oven to 350F.
2. Whisk the eggs, pumpkin, coconut oil, maple syrup, vanilla extract and almond butter in a large mixing bowl.
3. Sift the baking soda, cinnamon, coconut flour and pumpkin spice into the egg mixture and blend until well combined.
4. Pour the mixture in oven safe ramekins and bake in the center until the soufflé puffs up, around 25-35 minutes.

5. You can also turn this into a savory dish by replacing the sweet spices with savory ones like sage and black pepper.

# Mocha Bacon Brownies

*Makes: 12 brownies*

*Nutritional Info: (per serving)*

*Calories: 203*

*Total fat: 15g*

*Cholesterol: 54mg*

*Protein: 3g*

**Preparation Time: 15 minutes**

**Cooking Time: 30 minutes**

## Ingredients:

I. 4 ounces dark chocolate (70% or more)
II. ½ cup pure maple syrup
III. ½ cup coconut butter, melted and cooled
IV. 3 eggs
V. 2 tbsp strong coffee
VI. 2 slices baked bacon, chopped
VII. 2 tbsp fine coffee grinds
VIII. ½ cup unsweetened cocoa powder

## Method:

1. Preheat the oven to 375F.
2. Combine the melted dark chocolate, maple syrup, eggs and butter in a mixing bowl.
3. Sift the cocoa powder over the egg and chocolate mixture.
4. Add coffee grinds and strong coffee and blend.
5. Line a 9X9 inch square pan with parchment paper and add the brownie batter.
6. Top the batter with bacon pieces and bake for 25 minutes. Make sure you don't open the door of the oven in between or your brownies will become flat.

# Mint, Cream and Orange Melts

*Makes: 8 servings*

*Nutritional Info: (per serving)*

*Calories: 214*

*Total fat: 23g*

*Cholesterol: 0mg*

*Protein: 9g*

**Preparation Time: 15 minutes**

**Cooking Time: 0 minutes**

## Ingredients:

I. ½ cup coconut oil
II. ½ cup coconut manna
III. 2 tsp fresh mint, chopped
IV. 4 tsp pure maple syrup, divided
V. 2 tsp mint extract
VI. ½ tsp vanilla extract
VII. Zest of 1 orange

## Method:

1. Mix coconut milk and manna and blend into a smooth mixture.
2. In a separate bowl add vanilla extract, zest of orange and 2 tsp of maples syrup and mix.
3. Add fresh mint, mint extract and 2 tsp maple syrup in a bowl and mix well.
4. Combine all the three mixtures and refrigerate or freeze until set.

www.ingramcontent.com/pod-product-compliance
Lightning Source LLC
Chambersburg PA
CBHW080431290526
45791CB00008BA/2452